MedicalCenter.com

The Key Facts on Depression

Everything You Need to Know About Depression

-Usable Medical Information for the Patient-

By Patrick W. Nee

www.MedicalCenter.com

Published by:
MedicalCenter.com
96 Walter Street/ Suite 200
Boston, MA 02131, USA
Tel: 617-354-7722
www.MedicalCenter.com
manager@medicalcenter.com

Copyright © 2013 by PWN

"Key Facts" is a TradeMark.

All Rights are reserved under International, Pan-American, and Pan-Asian Conventions. No part of this book may be reproduced in any form without the written permission of the publisher. All rights vigorously enforced.

Table of Contents

Chapter 1: Introduction
    What is Depression?
    What are the Different Forms of Depression?

Chapter 2: Causes, Signs, and Symptoms of Depression
    What are the Causes of Depression?
    What are the Signs and Symptoms of Depression?
    What Illnesses Often Coexist with Depression?
    Who is at Risk for Depression?

Chapter 3: Diagnosis and Treatment of Depression
    How is Depression Diagnosed and Treated?
    Medications
        -How Should I Take the Medication?
        -What are the Side Effects of Antidepressants?
        -The FDA Warning on Antidepressants
    Psychotherapy
    Electroconvulsive Therapy and other Brain Stimulation Therapies
    What Efforts are Underway to Improve Treatment?

Chapter 4: Depression in Women

How Do Women Experience Depression?

What Causes Depression in Women?

- Genetics
- Chemicals and Hormones
- Premenstrual Dysphoric Disorder
- Postpartum Depression
- Menopause
- Stress

What Illnesses Often Coexist with Depression in Women?

- Depression and Pregnancy

Chapter 5: Depression in Men

How do Men Experience Depression?

What Causes Depression in Men?

Chapter 6: Depression in Adolescents

How do Adolescents Experience Depression?

How Can I Recognize Adolescent Depression?

- Be Aware of the Risk for Teen Depression
- Know the Symptoms of Depression
- Bring Your Teen to a Health Care Provider
- Identify Your Teen's Depression Early

Chapter 7: Depression in the Elderly

How do the Elderly Experience Depression?

What Causes Depression in the Elderly?

What are the Symptoms of Depression in the Elderly?

What is the Treatment for Depression in the Elderly?

-Outlook (Prognosis)

-When to Contact a Medical Professional

Chapter 8: Coping with Depression

How Can I Help Myself if I am Depressed?

-Self Help Tips

Where Can I Go for Help?

-Mental Health Resources

How Can I Help a Loved One Who is Depressed?

-Tips to Help Your Loved One

What if I or Someone I Know is in Crisis?

Chapter 1: Introduction

What is Depression?

Everyone occasionally feels blue or sad. But these feelings are usually short-lived and pass within a couple of days. When you have depression, it interferes with daily life and causes pain for both you and those who care about you. Depression is a common but serious illness.
Many people with a depressive illness never seek treatment. But the majority, even those with the most severe depression, can get better with treatment. Medications, psychotherapies, and other methods can effectively treat people with depression.

What are the different forms of Depression?

There are several forms of depressive disorders.

Major depressive disorder, or major depression, is characterized by a combination of symptoms that interfere with a person's ability to work, sleep, study, eat, and enjoy once-pleasurable activities. Major depression is disabling and prevents a person from functioning normally. Some people may experience only a single episode within their lifetime, but more often a person may have multiple episodes. Depression is a common but serious illness. Most who experience depression need treatment to get better.

Dysthymic disorder, or dysthymia, is characterized by long-term (2 years or longer) symptoms that may not be severe enough to disable a person but can prevent normal functioning or feeling well. People with dysthymia may also experience one or more episodes of major depression during their lifetimes.

Minor depression is characterized by having symptoms for 2 weeks or longer that do not meet full criteria for major depression. Without treatment, people with minor depression are at high risk for developing major depressive disorder. Some forms of depression are slightly different, or they may develop under unique circumstances. However, not everyone agrees on how to characterize and define these forms of depression. They include:
- Psychotic depression, which occurs when a person has severe depression plus some form of psychosis, such as having disturbing false beliefs or a break with

reality (delusions), or hearing or seeing upsetting things that others cannot hear or see (hallucinations).

- <u>Postpartum depression</u>, which is much more serious than the "baby blues" that many women experience after giving birth, when hormonal and physical changes and the new responsibility of caring for a newborn can be overwhelming. It is estimated that 10 to 15 percent of women experience postpartum depression after giving birth.

- <u>Seasonal affective disorder (SAD)</u>, which is characterized by the onset of depression during the winter months, when there is less natural sunlight. The depression generally lifts during spring and summer. SAD may be effectively treated with light therapy, but nearly half of those with SAD do not get better with light therapy alone. Antidepressant medication and psychotherapy can reduce SAD symptoms, either alone or in combination with light therapy.

Bipolar disorder, also called manic-depressive illness, is not as common as major depression or dysthymia. Bipolar disorder is characterized by cycling mood changes—from extreme highs (e.g., mania) to extreme lows (e.g., depression).

Chapter 2: Causes, Signs, and Symptoms of Depression

What are the Causes of Depression?

Several factors, or a combination of factors, may contribute to depression.

- <u>Genes</u>—people with a family history of depression may be more likely to develop it than those whose families do not have the illness.
- <u>Brain chemistry</u>—people with depression have different brain chemistry than those without the illness.
- <u>Stress</u>—loss of a loved one, a difficult relationship, or any stressful situation may trigger depression.

Most likely, depression is caused by a combination of genetic, biological, environmental, and psychological factors. Depressive illnesses are disorders of the brain. Brain-imaging technologies, such as magnetic resonance imaging (MRI), have shown that the brains of people who have depression look different than those of people without depression. The parts of the brain involved in mood, thinking, sleep, appetite, and behavior appear different. But these images do not reveal why the depression has occurred. They also cannot be used to diagnose depression.

Some types of depression tend to run in families. However, depression can occur in people without family histories of depression too. Scientists are studying certain genes that may make some people more prone to depression. Some genetics research indicates that risk for depression results from the influence of several genes acting together with environmental or other factors. In addition, trauma, loss of a loved one, a difficult relationship, or any stressful situation may trigger a depressive episode. Other depressive episodes may occur with or without an obvious trigger.

What are the Signs and Symptoms of Depression?

People with depressive illnesses do not all experience the same symptoms. The severity, frequency, and duration of symptoms vary depending on the individual and his or her particular illness.

Some common signs and symptoms are:
- Persistent sad, anxious, or "empty" feelings
- Feelings of hopelessness or pessimism
- Feelings of guilt, worthlessness, or helplessness

- Irritability, restlessness
- Loss of interest in activities or hobbies once pleasurable, including sex
- Fatigue and decreased energy
- Difficulty concentrating, remembering details, and making decisions
- Insomnia, early-morning wakefulness, or excessive sleeping
- Overeating, or appetite loss
- Thoughts of suicide, suicide attempts
- Aches or pains, headaches, cramps, or digestive problems that do not ease even with treatment.

What Illnesses Often Co-Exist with Depression?

Other illnesses may come on before depression, cause it, or be a consequence of it. But depression and other illnesses interact differently in different people. In any case, co-occurring illnesses need to be diagnosed and treated. Anxiety disorders, such as post-traumatic stress disorder (PTSD), obsessive-compulsive disorder, panic disorder, social phobia, and generalized anxiety disorder, often accompany depression. PTSD can occur after a person experiences a terrifying event or ordeal, such as a violent assault, a natural disaster, an accident, terrorism or military combat. People experiencing PTSD are especially prone to having co-existing depression.

In a National Institute of Mental Health (NIMH)-funded study, researchers found that more than 40 percent of people with PTSD also had depression 4 months after the traumatic event.

Alcohol and other substance abuse or dependence may also co-exist with depression. Research shows that mood disorders and substance abuse commonly occur together. Depression also may occur with other serious medical illnesses such as heart disease, stroke, cancer, HIV/AIDS, diabetes, and Parkinson's disease. People who have depression along with another medical illness tend to have more severe symptoms of both depression and the medical illness, more difficulty adapting to their medical condition, and more medical costs than those who do not have co-existing depression. Treating the depression can also help improve the outcome of treating the co-occurring illness.

Who is at Risk for Depression?

Major depressive disorder is one of the most common mental disorders in the United States. Each year about 6.7% of U.S adults experience major depressive disorder. Women are 70 % more likely than men to experience depression during their lifetime. Non-Hispanic blacks are 40% less likely than non-Hispanic whites to experience depression during their lifetime. The average age of onset is 32 years old. Additionally, 3.3% of 13 to 18 year olds have experienced a seriously debilitating depressive disorder.

Chapter 3: Diagnosis and Treatment of Depression

How is Depression Diagnosed and Treated?

Depression, even the most severe cases, can be effectively treated. The earlier that treatment can begin, the more effective it is.

The first step to getting appropriate treatment is to visit a doctor or mental health specialist. Certain medications, and some medical conditions such as viruses or a thyroid disorder, can cause the same symptoms as depression. A doctor can rule out these possibilities by doing a physical exam, interview, and lab tests. If the doctor can find no medical condition that may be causing the depression, the next step is a psychological evaluation.

The doctor may refer you to a mental health professional, who should discuss with you any family history of depression or other mental disorder, and get a complete history of your symptoms. You should discuss when your symptoms started, how long they have lasted, how severe they are, and whether they have occurred before and if so, how they were treated. The mental health professional may also ask if you are using alcohol or drugs, and if you are thinking about death or suicide.

Other illnesses may come on before depression, cause it, or be a consequence of it. But depression and other illnesses interact differently in different people. In any case, co-occurring illnesses need to be diagnosed and treated.

Anxiety disorders, such as post-traumatic stress disorder (PTSD), obsessive-compulsive disorder, panic disorder, social phobia, and generalized anxiety disorder, often accompany depression. PTSD can occur after a person experiences a terrifying event or ordeal, such as a violent assault, a natural disaster, an accident, terrorism or military combat. People experiencing PTSD are especially prone to having co-existing depression.

Alcohol and other substance abuse or dependence may also co-exist with depression. Research shows that mood disorders and substance abuse commonly occur together. Depression also may occur with other serious medical illnesses such as heart disease, stroke, cancer, HIV/AIDS, diabetes, and Parkinson's disease. People who have depression along with another medical illness tend to have more severe symptoms of both depression and the medical illness, more difficulty adapting to their medical condition, and more medical costs than those who do not have co-existing depression. Treating the depression can also help improve the outcome of treating the co-occurring illness.

Medications

Antidepressants primarily work on brain chemicals called neurotransmitters, especially serotonin and norepinephrine. Other antidepressants work on the neurotransmitter dopamine. Scientists have found that these particular chemicals are involved in regulating mood, but they are unsure of the exact ways that they work. The latest information on medications for treating depression is available on the U.S. Food and Drug Administration (FDA) website www.fda.gov

Popular newer antidepressants

Some of the newest and most popular antidepressants are called selective serotonin reuptake inhibitors (SSRIs). Fluoxetine (Prozac), sertraline (Zoloft), escitalopram (Lexapro), paroxetine (Paxil), and citalopram (Celexa) are some of the most commonly prescribed SSRIs for depression. Most are available in generic versions. Serotonin and norepinephrine reuptake inhibitors (SNRIs) are similar to SSRIs and include venlafaxine (Effexor) and duloxetine (Cymbalta).

SSRIs and SNRIs tend to have fewer side effects than older antidepressants, but they sometimes produce headaches, nausea, jitters, or insomnia when people first start to take them. These symptoms tend to fade with time. Some people also experience sexual problems with SSRIs or SNRIs, which may be helped by adjusting the dosage or switching to another medication.

One popular antidepressant that works on dopamine is bupropion (Wellbutrin). Bupropion tends to have similar side effects as SSRIs and SNRIs, but it is less likely to cause sexual side effects. However, it can increase a person's risk for seizures.

Tricyclics

Tricyclics are older antidepressants. Tricyclics are powerful, but they are not used as much today because their potential side effects are more serious. They may affect the heart in people with heart conditions. They sometimes cause dizziness, especially in older adults. They also may cause drowsiness, dry mouth, and weight gain. These side effects can usually be corrected by changing the dosage or switching to another medication. However, tricyclics may be especially dangerous if taken in overdose. Tricyclics include imipramine and nortriptyline.

MAOIs

Monoamine oxidase inhibitors (MAOIs) are the oldest class of antidepressant medications. They can be especially effective in cases of "atypical" depression, such as when a person experiences increased appetite and the need for more sleep rather than decreased appetite and sleep. They also may help with anxious feelings or panic and other specific symptoms.

However, people who take MAOIs must avoid certain foods and beverages (including cheese and red wine) that contain a substance called tyramine. Certain medications, including some types of birth control pills, prescription pain relievers, cold and allergy medications, and herbal supplements, also should be avoided while taking an MAOI. These substances can interact with MAOIs to cause dangerous increases in blood pressure. The development of a new MAOI skin patch may help reduce these risks. If you are taking an MAOI, your doctor should give you a complete list of foods, medicines, and substances to avoid.

MAOIs can also react with SSRIs to produce a serious condition called "serotonin syndrome," which can cause confusion, hallucinations, increased sweating, muscle stiffness, seizures, changes in blood pressure or heart rhythm, and other potentially life-threatening conditions. MAOIs should not be taken with SSRIs.

HOW SHOULD I TAKE THE MEDICATION?

All antidepressants must be taken for at least 4 to 6 weeks before they have a full effect. You should continue to take the medication, even if you are feeling better, to prevent the depression from returning.

Medication should be stopped only under a doctor's supervision. Some medications need to be gradually stopped to give the body time to adjust. Although antidepressants are not habit-forming or addictive, suddenly ending an antidepressant can cause withdrawal symptoms or lead to a relapse of the depression. Some individuals, such as those with chronic or recurrent depression, may need to stay on the medication indefinitely.

In addition, if one medication does not work, you should consider trying another. NIMH-funded research has shown that people who did not get well after taking a first medication increased their chances of beating the depression after they switched to a different medication or added another medication to their existing one.

Sometimes stimulants, anti-anxiety medications, or other medications are used together with an antidepressant, especially if a person has a co-existing illness. However, neither anti-anxiety medications nor stimulants are effective against depression when taken alone, and both should be taken only under a doctor's close supervision.

WHAT ARE THE SIDE EFFECTS OF ANTIDEPRESSANTS?

Antidepressants may cause mild and often temporary side effects in some people, but usually they are not long-term. However, any unusual reactions or side effects that interfere with normal functioning or are persistent or troublesome should be reported to a doctor immediately.

The most common side effects associated with SSRIs and SNRIs include:

- Headache-usually temporary and will subside.
- Nausea-temporary and usually short-lived.
- Insomnia and nervousness (trouble falling asleep or waking often during the night)-may occur during the first few weeks but often subside over time or if the dose is reduced.
- Agitation (e.g., feeling jittery).
- Sexual problems-women can experience sexual problems including reduced sex drive and problems having and enjoying sex.

Tricyclic antidepressants also can cause side effects including:

- Dry mouth-it is helpful to drink plenty of water, chew gum, and clean teeth daily.
- Constipation-it is helpful to eat more bran cereals, prunes, fruits, and vegetables.
- Bladder problems-emptying the bladder may be difficult, and the urine stream may not be as strong as usual.
- Sexual problems-sexual functioning may change, and side effects are similar to those from SSRIs and SNRIs.
- Blurred vision-often passes soon and usually will not require a new corrective lenses prescription.
- Drowsiness during the day-usually passes soon, but driving or operating heavy machinery should be avoided while drowsiness occurs. These more sedating antidepressants are generally taken at bedtime to help sleep and minimize daytime drowsiness.

THE FDA WARNING ON ANTIDEPRESSANTS

Despite the relative safety and popularity of SSRIs and other antidepressants, studies have suggested that they may have unintentional effects on some people, especially adolescents and young adults. In 2004, the Food and Drug Administration (FDA) conducted a thorough review of published and unpublished controlled clinical trials of antidepressants that involved nearly 4,400 children and adolescents. The review revealed that 4 percent of those taking antidepressants thought about or attempted suicide (although no suicides occurred), compared to 2 percent of those receiving placebos.

This information prompted the FDA, in 2005, to adopt a "black box" warning label on all antidepressant medications to alert the public about the potential increased risk of suicidal thinking or attempts in children and adolescents taking antidepressants. In 2007, the FDA proposed that makers of all antidepressant medications extend the warning to include young adults up through age 24. A "black box" warning is the most serious type of warning on prescription drug labeling.

The warning emphasizes that patients of all ages taking antidepressants should be closely monitored, especially during the initial weeks of treatment. Possible side effects to look for are worsening depression, suicidal thinking or behavior, or any unusual changes in behavior such as sleeplessness, agitation, or withdrawal from normal social situations. The warning adds that families and caregivers should also be told of the need for close monitoring and report any changes to the doctor.

Results of a comprehensive review of pediatric trials conducted between 1988 and 2006 suggested that the benefits of antidepressant medications likely outweigh their risks to children and adolescents with major depression and anxiety disorders.30 The study was funded in part by NIMH.

Also, the FDA issued a warning that combining an SSRI or SNRI antidepressant with one of the commonly-used "triptan" medications for migraine headache could cause a life-threatening "serotonin syndrome," marked by agitation, hallucinations, elevated body temperature, and rapid changes in blood pressure. Although most dramatic in the case of the MAOIs, newer antidepressants may also be associated with potentially dangerous interactions with other medications.

What about St. John's wort?

The extract from the herb St. John's wort (Hypericum perforatum) has been used for centuries in many folk and herbal remedies. Today in Europe, it is used extensively to treat mild to moderate depression. In the United States, it is one of the top-selling botanical products.

In an 8-week trial involving 340 patients diagnosed with major depression, St. John's wort was compared to a common SSRI and a placebo (sugar pill). The trial found that St. John's wort was no more effective than the placebo in treating major depression.31 However, use of St. John's wort for minor or moderate depression may be more effective. Its use in the treatment of depression remains under study.

St. John's wort can interact with other medications, including those used to control HIV infection. In 2000, the FDA issued a Public Health Advisory letter stating that the herb may interfere with certain medications used to treat heart disease, depression, seizures, certain cancers, and those used to prevent organ transplant rejection. The herb also may interfere with the effectiveness of oral contraceptives. Consult with your doctor before taking any herbal supplement.

Psychotherapy

Several types of psychotherapy—or "talk therapy"—can help people with depression.

Two main types of psychotherapies—cognitive-behavioral therapy (CBT) and interpersonal therapy (IPT)—are effective in treating depression. CBT helps people with depression restructure negative thought patterns. Doing so helps people interpret their environment and interactions with others in a positive and realistic way. It may also help you recognize things that may be contributing to the depression and help you change behaviors that may be making the depression worse. IPT helps people understand and work through troubled relationships that may cause their depression or make it worse.

For mild to moderate depression, psychotherapy may be the best option. However, for severe depression or for certain people, psychotherapy may not be enough. For teens, a combination of medication and psychotherapy may be the most effective approach to treating major depression and reducing the chances of it coming back. Another study looking at depression treatment among older adults found that people who responded to initial treatment of medication and IPT were less likely to have recurring depression if they continued their combination treatment for at least 2 years.

Electroconvulsive Therapy and Other Brain Stimulation Therapies

For cases in which medication and/or psychotherapy does not help relieve a person's treatment-resistant depression, electroconvulsive therapy (ECT) may be useful. ECT, formerly known as "shock therapy," once had a bad reputation. But in recent years, it has greatly improved and can provide relief for people with severe depression who have not been able to feel better with other treatments. Before ECT begins, a patient is put under brief anesthesia and given a muscle relaxant. He or she sleeps through the treatment and does not consciously feel the electrical impulses. Within 1 hour after the treatment session, which takes only a few minutes, the patient is awake and alert. A person typically will undergo ECT several times a week, and often will need to take an antidepressant or other medication along with the ECT treatments. Although some people will need only a few courses of ECT, others may need maintenance ECT—usually once a week at first, then gradually decreasing to monthly treatments. Ongoing NIMH-supported ECT research is aimed at developing personalized maintenance ECT schedules.

ECT may cause some side effects, including confusion, disorientation, and memory loss. Usually these side effects are short-term, but sometimes they can linger. Newer methods of administering the treatment have reduced the memory loss and other cognitive difficulties associated with

ECT. Research has found that after 1 year of ECT treatments, most patients showed no adverse cognitive effects. Nevertheless, patients always provide informed consent before receiving ECT, ensuring that they understand the potential benefits and risks of the treatment.

Other more recently introduced types of brain stimulation therapies used to treat severe depression include vagus nerve stimulation (VNS), and repetitive transcranial magnetic stimulation (rTMS). These methods are not yet commonly used, but research has suggested that they show promise.

What Efforts are Underway to Improve Treatment?

Researchers are looking for ways to better understand, diagnose and treat depression among all groups of people. New possible treatments, such as faster-acting antidepressants, are being tested that give hope to those who live with difficult-to-treat depression. Researchers are studying the risk factors for depression and how it affects the brain. NIMH continues to fund cutting-edge research into this debilitating disorder.

Chapter 4: Depression in Women

How Do Women Experience Depression?

Depression is more common among women than among men. Biological, life cycle, hormonal, and psychosocial factors that women experience may be linked to women's higher depression rate. Researchers have shown that hormones directly affect the brain chemistry that controls emotions and mood. For example, women are especially vulnerable to developing postpartum depression after giving birth, when hormonal and physical changes and the new responsibility of caring for a newborn can be overwhelming. Some women may also have a severe form of premenstrual syndrome (PMS) called premenstrual dysphoric disorder (PMDD). PMDD is associated with the hormonal changes that typically occur around ovulation and before menstruation begins.

During the transition into menopause, some women experience an increased risk for depression. In addition, osteoporosis—bone thinning or loss—may be associated with depression. Scientists are exploring all of these potential connections and how the cyclical rise and fall of estrogen and other hormones may affect a woman's brain chemistry.

Finally, many women face the additional stresses of work and home responsibilities, caring for children and aging parents, abuse, poverty, and relationship strains. It is still unclear, though, why some women faced with enormous challenges develop depression, while others with similar challenges do not.

What Causes Depression in Women?

Scientists are examining many potential causes for and contributing factors to women's increased risk for depression. It is likely that genetic, biological, chemical, hormonal, environmental, psychological, and social factors all intersect to contribute to depression.

GENETICS

If a woman has a family history of depression, she may be more at risk of developing the illness. However, this is not a hard and fast rule. Depression can occur in women without family histories of depression, and women from families with a history of depression may not develop depression themselves. Genetics research indicates that the risk for developing depression likely involves the combination of multiple genes with environmental or other factors.

CHEMICALS AND HORMONES

Brain chemistry appears to be a significant factor in depressive disorders. Modern brain-imaging technologies, such as magnetic resonance imaging (MRI), have shown that the brains of people suffering from depression look different than those of people without depression. The parts of the brain responsible for regulating mood, thinking, sleep, appetite and behavior don't appear to be functioning normally. In addition, important neurotransmitters-chemicals that brain cells use to communicate-appear to be out of balance. But these images do not reveal WHY the depression has occurred.

Scientists are also studying the influence of female hormones, which change throughout life. Researchers have shown that hormones directly affect the brain chemistry that controls emotions and mood. Specific times during a woman's life are of particular interest, including puberty; the times before menstrual periods; before, during, and just after pregnancy (postpartum); and just prior to and during menopause (perimenopause).

PREMENSTRUAL DYSPHORIC DISORDER

Some women may be susceptible to a severe form of premenstrual syndrome called premenstrual dysphoric disorder (PMDD). Women affected by PMDD typically experience depression, anxiety, irritability and mood swings the week before menstruation, in such a way that interferes with their normal functioning. Women with debilitating PMDD do not necessarily have unusual hormone changes, but they do have different responses to these changes. They may also have a history of other mood disorders and differences in brain chemistry that cause them to be more sensitive to menstruation-related hormone changes. Scientists are exploring how the cyclical rise and fall of estrogen and other hormones may affect the brain chemistry that is associated with depressive illness.

POSTPARTUM DEPRESSION

Women are particularly vulnerable to depression after giving birth, when hormonal and physical changes and the new responsibility of caring for a newborn can be overwhelming. Many new mothers experience a brief episode of mild mood changes known as the "baby blues," but some will suffer from postpartum depression, a much more serious condition that requires active treatment and emotional support for the new mother. One study found that postpartum women are at an increased risk for several mental disorders, including depression, for several months after childbirth.

Some studies suggest that women who experience postpartum depression often have had prior depressive episodes. Some experience it during their pregnancies, but it often goes undetected. Research suggests that visits to the doctor may be good opportunities for screening for depression both during pregnancy and in the postpartum period.

MENOPAUSE

Hormonal changes increase during the transition between premenopause to menopause. While some women may transition into menopause without any problems with mood, others experience an increased risk for depression. This seems to occur even among women without a history of depression. However, depression becomes less common for women during the post-menopause period.

STRESS

Stressful life events such as trauma, loss of a loved one, a difficult relationship or any stressful situation-whether welcome or unwelcome-often occur before a depressive episode. Additional work and home responsibilities, caring for children and aging parents, abuse, and poverty also may trigger a depressive episode. Evidence suggests that women respond differently than men to these events, making them more prone to depression. In fact, research indicates that women respond in such a way that prolongs their feelings of stress more so than men, increasing the risk for depression. However, it is unclear why some women faced with enormous challenges develop depression, and some with similar challenges do not.

What Illnesses Often Coexist with Depression in Women?

Depression often coexists with other illnesses that may precede the depression, follow it, cause it, be a consequence of it, or a combination of these. It is likely that the interplay between depression and other illnesses differs for every person and situation. Regardless, these other coexisting illnesses need to be diagnosed and treated.

Depression often coexists with eating disorders such as anorexia nervosa, bulimia nervosa and others, especially among women. Anxiety disorders, such as post-traumatic stress disorder (PTSD), obsessive-compulsive disorder, panic disorder, social phobia and generalized anxiety disorder, also sometimes accompany depression. Women are more prone than men to having a coexisting anxiety disorder. Women suffering from PTSD, which can result after a person endures a terrifying ordeal or event, are especially prone to having depression.

Although more common among men than women, alcohol and substance abuse or dependence may occur at the same time as depression. Research has indicated that among both sexes, the coexistence of mood disorders and substance abuse is common among the U.S. population.

Depression also often coexists with other serious medical illnesses such as heart disease, stroke, cancer, HIV/AIDS, diabetes, Parkinson's disease, thyroid problems and multiple sclerosis, and may even make symptoms of the illness worse. Studies have shown that both women and men who have depression in addition to a serious medical illness tend to have more severe symptoms of both illnesses. They also have more difficulty adapting to their medical condition, and more medical costs than those who do not have coexisting depression. Research has shown that treating the depression along with the coexisting illness will help ease both conditions.

DEPRESSION AND PREGNANCY

Is it safe to take antidepressant medication during pregnancy?

At one time, doctors assumed that pregnancy was accompanied by a natural feeling of well being, and that depression during pregnancy was rare, or never occurred at all. However, recent studies have shown that women can have depression while pregnant, especially if they have a prior history of the illness. In fact, a majority of women with a history of depression will likely relapse during pregnancy if they stop taking their antidepressant medication either prior to conception or early in the pregnancy, putting both mother and baby at risk.

However, antidepressant medications do pass across the placental barrier, potentially exposing the developing fetus to the medication. Some research suggests the use of SSRIs during pregnancy is associated with miscarriage and/or birth defects, but other studies do not support this. Some studies have indicated that fetuses exposed to SSRIs during the third trimester may be born with "withdrawal" symptoms such as breathing problems, jitteriness, irritability, difficulty feeding, or hypoglycemia. In 2004, the U.S. Food and Drug Administration (FDA) issued a warning against the use of

SSRIs in the late third trimester, suggesting that clinicians gradually taper expectant mothers off SSRIs in the third trimester to avoid any ill effects on the baby.

Although some studies suggest that exposure to SSRIs in pregnancy may have adverse effects on the infant, generally they are mild and short-lived, and no deaths have been reported. On the flip side, women who stop taking their antidepressant medication during pregnancy increase their risk for developing depression again and may put both themselves and their infant at risk.

In light of these mixed results, women and their doctors need to consider the potential risks and benefits to both mother and fetus of taking an antidepressant during pregnancy, and make decisions based on individual needs and circumstances. In some cases, a woman and her doctor may decide to taper her antidepressant dose during the last month of pregnancy to minimize the newborn's withdrawal symptoms, and after delivery, return to a full dose during the vulnerable postpartum period.

Is it safe to take antidepressant medication while breastfeeding?

Antidepressants are excreted in breast milk, usually in very small amounts. The amount an infant receives is usually so small that it does not register in blood tests. Few problems are seen among infants nursing from mothers who are taking antidepressants. However, as with antidepressant use during pregnancy, both the risks and benefits to the mother and infant should be taken into account when deciding whether to take an antidepressant while breastfeeding.

Chapter 5: Depression in Men

How do Men Experience Depression?

Men often experience depression differently than women. While women with depression are more likely to have feelings of sadness, worthlessness, and excessive guilt, men are more likely to be very tired, irritable, lose interest in once-pleasurable activities, and have difficulty sleeping. Men may be more likely than women to turn to alcohol or drugs when they are depressed. They also may become frustrated, discouraged, irritable, angry, and sometimes abusive. Some men throw themselves into their work to avoid talking about their depression with family or friends, or behave recklessly. And although more women attempt suicide, many more men die by suicide in the United States. In America alone, more than 6 million men have depression each year.

What Causes Depression in Men?

Several factors may contribute to depression in men.

- <u>Genes</u>—men with a family history of depression may be more likely to develop it than those whose family members do not have the illness.

- <u>Brain chemistry and hormones</u>—the brains of people with depression look different on scans than those of people without the illness. Also, the hormones that control emotions and mood can affect brain chemistry.
- <u>Stress</u>—loss of a loved one, a difficult relationship or any stressful situation may trigger depression in some men.

Most of the time, it is likely a combination of these factors.

Chapter 6: Depression in Adolescents

How do Adolescents Experience Depression?

Children who develop depression often continue to have episodes as they enter adulthood. Children who have depression also are more likely to have other more severe illnesses in adulthood.

A child with depression may pretend to be sick, refuse to go to school, cling to a parent, or worry that a parent may die. Older children may sulk, get into trouble at school, be negative and irritable, and feel misunderstood. Because these signs may be viewed as normal mood swings typical of children as they move through developmental stages, it may be difficult to accurately diagnose a young person with depression.

Before puberty, boys and girls are equally likely to develop depression. By age 15, however, girls are twice as likely as boys to have had a major depressive episode.

Depression during the teen years comes at a time of great personal change—when boys and girls are forming an identity apart from their parents, grappling with gender issues and emerging sexuality, and making independent decisions for the first time in their lives. Depression in adolescence frequently co-occurs with other disorders such as anxiety, eating disorders, or substance abuse. It can also lead to increased risk for suicide.

An National Institute of Mental Health (NIMH)-funded clinical trial of 439 adolescents with major depression found that a combination of medication and psychotherapy was the most effective treatment option. Other NIMH-funded researchers are developing and testing ways to prevent suicide in children and adolescents.

Childhood depression often persists, recurs, and continues into adulthood, especially if left untreated.

How can I Recognize Adolescent Depression?

About 1 in 5 teenagers have depression at some point. Your teen may be depressed if they are feeling sad, blue, unhappy, or down in the dumps. Depression is a serious problem, even more so if these feelings have taken over their life.

BE AWARE OF THE RISK FOR TEEN DEPRESSION

Your teen is more at risk for depression if:
- Mood disorders run in your family

- They experience a stressful life event like a death in the family, divorcing parents, bullying, a break up with a boyfriend or girlfriend, or failing in school
- They have low self-esteem and are very critical of themselves
- Your teen is a girl. Teen girls are twice as likely as boys to have depression.
- Your teen has trouble being social
- Your teen has learning disabilities
- Your teen has a chronic illness
- There are family problems or problems with their parents

KNOW THE SYMPTOMS OF DEPRESSION

If your teen is depressed, you may see some of the following common symptoms of depression. If these symptoms last for 2 weeks or longer, talk to your teen's doctor.

- Frequent irritability with sudden bursts of anger
- More sensitive to criticism
- Complaints of headaches, stomachaches or other body problems. Your teen may go to the nurse's office at school a lot.
- Withdrawal from people like parents or some friends

- Not enjoying activities they usually like
- Feeling tired for much of the day
- Sad or blue feelings most of the time

Notice changes in your teen's daily routines that can be a sign of depression. Your teen's daily routines can change when they are depressed. You may notice that your teen has:

- Trouble sleeping or is sleeping more than normal
- A change in eating habits, such as not being hungry or eating more than usual
- A hard time concentrating
- Problems making decisions

Notice changes in your teen's behavior that could be a sign of depression. They could be having problems at home or school.

- Drop in school grades, attendance, not doing homework
- High-risk behaviors, such as reckless driving, unsafe sex, or shoplifting
- Pulling away from family and friends and spends more time alone
- Drinking or using drugs

Teens with depression may also have:

- Anxiety disorders
- Attention deficit hyperactivity disorder (ADHD)

- Bipolar disorder
- Eating disorders (such as bulimia or anorexia)

BRING YOUR TEEN TO A HEALTH CARE PROVIDER

If you are worried that your teen is depressed, see a health care provider. The health care provider may perform a physical exam and order blood tests to make sure your teen doesn't have a medical problem.

The health care provider should talk to your teen about:

- Their sadness, irritability, or loss of interest in normal activities
- Signs of other mental health problems, such as anxiety, mania, or schizophrenia
- Risk of suicide or other violence -- whether your teen is a danger to him or herself or others

The health care provider should ask about drug or alcohol abuse. Depressed teens are at risk for:

- Heavy drinking
- Regular marijuana (pot) smoking
- Other drug use

The health care provider may speak with other family members or your teen's teachers. These people can often help identify signs of depression in teenagers.

Be alert to any signs of suicide plans. Notice if your teen is:
- Giving possessions to others
- Saying good bye to family and friends
- Talking about dying or committing suicide
- Writing about dying or suicide
- Having a personality change
- Taking big risks
- Withdrawing and wanting to be alone

Call your health care provider or a suicide hotline right away if you are worried that your teen is thinking about suicide. Never ignore a suicide threat or attempt.

Call 1-800-SUICIDE or 1-800-999-9999. You can call 24/7 anywhere in the United States.

IDENTIFY YOUR TEEN'S DEPRESSION EARLY

Most teenagers feel down sometimes. Having support and good coping skills helps teens through down periods.

Talk with your teen frequently to check in with them. Ask them about their feelings. Talking about depression will not make the situation worse, and may help them to get help sooner.

Get your teen professional help to deal with low moods. Treating depression early may help them feel better sooner, and may prevent or delay future episodes.

Chapter 7: Depression in the Elderly

How do the Elderly Experience Depression?

Depression is not a normal part of aging. Studies show that most seniors feel satisfied with their lives, despite having more illnesses or physical problems. However, when older adults do have depression, it may be overlooked because seniors may show different, less obvious symptoms. They may be less likely to experience or admit to feelings of sadness or grief.

Sometimes it can be difficult to distinguish grief from major depression. Grief after loss of a loved one is a normal reaction to the loss and generally does not require professional mental health treatment. However, grief that is complicated and lasts for a very long time following a loss may require treatment. Researchers continue to study the relationship between complicated grief and major depression. Older adults also may have more medical conditions such as heart disease, stroke, or cancer, which may cause depressive symptoms. Or they may be taking medications with side effects that contribute to depression. Some older adults may experience what doctors call vascular depression, also called arteriosclerotic depression or subcortical ischemic depression. Vascular depression may result when blood vessels become less flexible and harden over time, becoming constricted. Such hardening of vessels prevents normal blood flow to the body's organs, including the brain. Those with vascular depression may have, or be at risk for, co-existing heart disease or stroke.

Although many people assume that the highest rates of suicide are among young people, older white males age 85 and older actually have the highest suicide rate in the United States. Many have a depressive illness that their doctors are not aware of, even though many of these suicide victims visit their doctors within 1 month of their deaths.

Most older adults with depression improve when they receive treatment with an antidepressant, psychotherapy, or a combination of both. Research has shown that medication alone and combination treatment are both effective in reducing depression in older adults. Psychotherapy alone also can be effective in helping older adults stay free of depression, especially among those with minor depression. Psychotherapy is particularly useful for those who are unable or unwilling to take antidepressant medication.

What Causes Depression in the Elderly?

In the elderly, a number of life changes can increase the risk for depression, or make existing depression worse. Some of these changes are:

- A move from home, such as to a retirement facility
- Chronic illness or pain
- Children moving away
- Spouse or close friends passing away
- Loss of independence (for example, problems getting around or caring for oneself)

Depression can also be related to a physical illness, such as:

- Thyroid disorders
- Parkinson's disease
- Heart disease
- Cancer
- Stroke
- Dementia (such as Alzheimer's disease)

Overuse of alcohol or certain medications (such as sleep aids) can make depression worse.

What are the Symptoms of Depression in the Elderly?

Many of the usual symptoms of depression may be seen. However, depression in the elderly may be hard to detect. Common symptoms such as fatigue, appetite loss, and trouble sleeping can be part of the aging process or a physical illness. As a result, early depression may be ignored, or confused with other conditions that are common in the elderly.

What is the Treatment for Depression in the Elderly?

The first steps of treatment are to:

- Treat any illness that may be causing the symptoms
- Stop taking any medications that may be making symptoms worse
- Avoid alcohol and sleep aids

If these steps do not help, medications to treat depression and talk therapy often help.

Doctors often prescribe lower doses of antidepressants to older people, and increase the dose more slowly than in younger adults.

To better manage depression at home, you should:

- Exercise regularly, if your doctor says it is ok.
- Surround yourself with caring, positive people and fun activities.
- Learn good sleeping habits.
- Learn to watch for the early signs of depression, and know how to react if these occur.
- Drink less alcohol and do not use illegal drugs.
- Talk about your feelings with someone you trust.
- Take medications correctly and discuss any side effects with your doctor.

OUTLOOK (PROGNOSIS)

Depression often responds to treatment. The outcome is usually better for people who have access to social services, family, and friends who can help them stay active and engaged.

The most worrisome complication of depression is suicide. Men make up most suicides among the elderly. Divorced or widowed men are at the highest risk.

Families should pay close attention to elderly relatives who are depressed and live alone.

WHEN TO CONTACT A MEDICAL PROFESSIONAL

Call your health care provider if you feel persistently sad, worthless, or hopeless, or if you cry often. Also call if you are having trouble coping with stresses in your life and want to be referred for talk therapy.

Go to the nearest emergency room or call your local emergency number (such as 911) if you are thinking about suicide (taking your own life).

If you are caring for an aging family member and think they may have depression, contact their health care provider.

Chapter 8: Coping with Depression

How Can I Help Myself if I am Depressed?

If you have depression, you may feel exhausted, helpless, and hopeless. It may be extremely difficult to take any action to help yourself. But as you begin to recognize your depression and begin treatment, you will start to feel better.

SELF-HELP TIPS

- Do not wait too long to get evaluated or treated. There is research showing the longer one waits, the greater the impairment can be down the road. Try to see a professional as soon as possible.
- Try to be active and exercise. Go to a movie, a ballgame, or another event or activity that you once enjoyed.
- Set realistic goals for yourself.
- Break up large tasks into small ones, set some priorities and do what you can as you can.
- Try to spend time with other people and confide in a trusted friend or relative. Try not to isolate yourself, and let others help you.
- Expect your mood to improve gradually, not immediately. Do not expect to suddenly "snap out of"

your depression. Often during treatment for depression, sleep and appetite will begin to improve before your depressed mood lifts.
- Postpone important decisions, such as getting married or divorced or changing jobs, until you feel better. Discuss decisions with others who know you well and have a more objective view of your situation.
- Remember that positive thinking will replace negative thoughts as your depression responds to treatment.
- Continue to educate yourself about depression.

Where Can I Go for Help?

If you are unsure where to go for help, ask your family doctor. Others who can help are listed below.

MENTAL HEALTH RESOURCES
- Mental health specialists, such as psychiatrists, psychologists, social workers, or mental health counselors
- Health maintenance organizations
- Community mental health centers
- Hospital psychiatry departments and outpatient clinics

- Mental health programs at universities or medical schools
- State hospital outpatient clinics
- Family services, social agencies, or clergy
- Peer support groups
- Private clinics and facilities
- Employee assistance programs
- Local medical and/or psychiatric societies
- You can also check the phone book under "mental health," "health," "social services," "hotlines," or "physicians" for phone numbers and addresses. An emergency room doctor also can provide temporary help and can tell you where and how to get further help.

How Can I Help a Loved One Who is Depressed?

If you know someone who is depressed, it affects you too. The most important thing you can do is help your friend or relative get a diagnosis and treatment. You may need to make an appointment and go with him or her to see the doctor. Encourage your loved one to stay in treatment, or to seek different treatment if no improvement occurs after 6 to 8 weeks.

TIPS TO HELP YOUR LOVED ONE

- Offer emotional support, understanding, patience, and encouragement.
- Talk to him or her, and listen carefully.
- Never dismiss feelings, but point out realities and offer hope.
- Never ignore comments about suicide, and report them to your loved one's therapist or doctor.
- Invite your loved one out for walks, outings and other activities. Keep trying if he or she declines, but don't push him or her to take on too much too soon.
- Provide assistance in getting to the doctor's appointments.
- Remind your loved one that with time and treatment, the depression will lift.

What if I or Someone I Know is in Crisis?

If you are thinking about harming yourself, or know someone who is, tell someone who can help immediately.

- Do not leave your friend or relative alone, and do not isolate yourself.

- Call your doctor.
- Call 911 or go to a hospital emergency room to get immediate help, or ask a friend or family member to help you do these things.
- Call the toll-free, 24-hour hotline of the National Suicide Prevention Lifeline at 1-800-273-TALK (1-800-273-8255); TTY: 1-800-799-4TTY (4889) to talk to a trained counselor

Other MedicalCenter.com Publications

The Key Facts on Arthritis

The Key Facts on Breast Cancer

The Key Facts on Medicare

The Key Facts on Cancer Types

The Key Facts on Cancer Treatment

The Key Facts on Cancer Risk Factors and Causes

The Key Facts on Cancer Prevention

The Key Facts on Cancer Detection & Diagnosis

The Key Facts on Coping With Cancer & Cancer Resources

The Key Facts on Alzheimer's Disease

The Key Facts on Caring For Someone With Alzheimer's Disease

The Key Facts on Obesity

The Key Facts on Diabetes

The Key Facts on Drug Abuse

The Key Facts on Attention Deficit Hyperactivity Disorder (ADHD)

All Titles Can Be Found at

www.Amazon.com

www.MedicalCenter.com

www.ingramcontent.com/pod-product-compliance
Lightning Source LLC
Chambersburg PA
CBHW071632170526
45166CB00003B/1306